Understanding Your Chakras and Aura for Beginners

Cindy Walker

The information contained in this book is intended to be educational and not for diagnosis, prescription, or treatment of any health disorder whatsoever. This information should not replace consultation with a competent health professional. The content of this book is intended to be used as an adjunct to a rational and responsible healthcare program prescribed by a professional healthcare provider. The author is in no way liable for any misuse of the material.

Cindy Walker

DEDICATION

For Love

This book is filled with information to give you a basic understanding of our internal energy system. It breaks down aura color and why it is important to be able to see auras. I have included tricks and methods to clean your aura that are practical and simple to apply every single day. You will get an understanding of how to sense, cleanse, and balance your internal energy starting today so that you can start attracting the things that you have always needed and desired! Let's get busy!

TABLE OF CONTENTS

THE CONCEPT OF UNIVERSAL ENERGY

Everything in the universe is connected: people, events, nature, even places. How? ENERGY! We are all full of energy that we pass along. The world and people around us are pulsating with an internal and external energy that we can pick up. We are miniscule drops of water in a vast ocean of universal energy. Some call this energy the universal mind. Have you ever wondered why no matter how hard you try you cannot achieve your goals? Nothing seems to go right for you? You cannot maintain the relationships you would like? Well my friends, it may be your own fault. Sorry to say, but your own negative energy may be the only thing standing in your way. Your own negative thought processes may be repelling what you want. No, it's probably not bad luck; it may be as simple as fixing your internal flow of energy. It may be as easy as cleansing your aura and freshening up your thoughts.

A brief explanation of what is called the law of attraction:

Everything and everyone in the universe is made up of energy.

Ideas and thoughts leave an energy trail.

What you think about, focus on, and put your energy into, you acquire; sometimes in excess.

Your emotions and feelings are energy that works like a magnet, the universal energy matches this energy by sending equal, echoing energy.

Now, you may already have conquered positive thinking. You may be doing all of the right exercises, using positive affirmations, visualizing the right things, and still not getting what it is that you want. This could be a career goal, a life's dream, or simply looking for love. What the heck is going on here?

Well, we have to remember a few things.

1. Our conscious brain is not always in tune with our spiritual mind. The two forms of energy must be in line and in agreement. Sometimes the spiritual mind knows better than our conscious mind.
2. Sometimes our spiritual and conscious mind are on a different time schedule than the universe. It is all about timing.
3. Our own internal energy flow has to be functioning at its best. It has to be free flowing and clean.

This is the one thing we have control over entirely. This is where the answer to our "problems" usually lies. We have the ability to cleanse our aura and allow our energy to flow freely throughout our spiritual body. Bad energy needs to be pushed out and blockages must be cleared. Some of those negative things are internal and some are external. Either way, you have the ability to fix it.

Our system is pumping and vibrating with universal energy. It flows through our chakras and out into our auras. Emotions and ideas change our energy flow and the type of energy that we have: be it positive or negative. When we clear blockages in our internal energy system and cleanse our auras, we will have positive ideas and exude positive energy. Guess what that attracts? You guessed it... positive things, events, and people.

The one thing that we can control is the type of energy we put off. You can have control over your life, relationships, and circumstances!

The balance of our energy system directly relates to how well we are able to use the law of attraction to our advantage. All we need to do is balance our internal energy. The key to doing this is to learn about auras and chakras, how to clear them and how to cleanse our energy. This is how we become the captain of our ship instead of the prisoner.

WHAT ARE CHAKRAS AND AURA?

Our world is alive with energy, quite literally. Everything in us and around us gives off energy of some sort . The atoms in our cells are configured so that each has both negative and positive charges, our own tiny batteries. Our physical bodies are constantly emitting and taking in energy. This energy is our life force. It effects our bodily functions, our emotions, and our spirituality. In turn, it is also affected by all of these things.

Chakras and auras are both ways that we can view, channel, access, and interact with this life energy. The power plants, or hubs, for our life energy are our chakras. These spinning wheels of light and energy are usually characterized as a row of colored circles that run from the head to the genitals. Chakras , in reality, are actually spinning vortexes of color and light that radiate from the center of the body, both through the front and the back.

There are seven main chakras.

Each channels the flow of energy through our beings. Chakras are the regulators and gate keepers of our life force. The level at which our chakras function is a reflection of how we choose to handle circumstances in life. Our thoughts, feelings, and how we generally view the world around us determine how open or closed our chakras are.

Chakras are an extension of our awareness.

They have more mass than auras, but less than the body. Even though they are part of our consciousness, chakras play a part in the physical processes of the body. Every chakra is linked with an endocrine gland. Each is also connected to a plexus, a network of nerves. Therefore, since every chakra covers a different area of the body, some physical ailments can be directly related to a chakra that is out of balance.

Every chakra vortex is made up of smaller vortexes. Each small vortex has a different rate of vibration and a different hue. They all combine together to make a certain tone and color when they are balanced. Each mini chakra is represents one of the many aspects of that chakra. If one thing is missing in your life, it can throw off the balance of the entire chakra. Not only does each chakra need to remain balanced, all of them must be in synch for the body, mind, and spirit to function optimally.

Our Seven Chakras:

- Starting at the base of the spine, near the tailbone you will find the Root Chakra. It is red in color. This chakra is responsible for feelings of security and survival (finances, food, and shelter). This chakra regulates the testes and the ovaries.

- Moving up along the spine, located right below the belly button you will find the Sacral Chakra. It is orange in color. This chakra is responsible for pleasure, sexuality, and happiness. It regulates the pancreas.

- Moving up along the spine to the upper abdomen you will find the Solar Plexus Chakra. It is yellow in color. This chakra is responsible for self-confidence, self-empowerment, and self-respect. It regulates the adrenals.

- Moving up to the center of the chest you will find the Heart Chakra. It is green in color. This chakra is responsible for love, joy, validation, and peace. It regulates the thymus.

- Moving up to the throat you will find the Throat Chakra. It is blue in color. This chakra is responsible for the ability to communicate and express thoughts and feelings. It regulates the thyroid.

- Moving up to the center of the forehead you will find the Third Eye Chakra. It is indigo in color. This chakra is responsible for clairvoyance, decision making, and imagination. It regulates the pituitary gland.

- Moving up to the top of the head you will find the Crown Chakra. It is violet in color and is responsible for spirituality (connection to your higher self), and beauty.

It is important to keep our chakras open and functioning at the highest level possible to achieve mental clarity, spirituality to the fullest, excellent health, and emotional wellness.

The chakras are essentially energy gates of the aura. They keep our auras luminous and vivid, and when they are in balance, they will keep us healthy and happy.

How chakras radiate energy into the aura

Our life-force energy is taken into the chakra via its inward bound vortex, where it is then transported into the center or main orb of the chakra. This central area is what we tend to define as the chakra. From there, it is transported through the meridians and the central channel (the current that passes the energy through each of the chakras vertically). As life-energy flows through the body, it is picked up by each persons' DNA and passed along to the nervous and endocrine systems. At the same time, our DNA is emitting the energy all around the outside of the body, creating the aura.

Auras are our own personal energy field. The world and people around us are affected by the energy of our aura.

Auras can actually be seen as a "glowing egg" of color, glowing around the human body. The color of one's aura is determined by the strongest chakras, although, the color is a mixture of all your chakra light energy. Everyone's aura can be seen as any one of the colors in the rainbow. They appear as different hues and shades, each one having a different meaning regarding emotion, spirituality, and health.

Auras are comprised of an equal amount of layers, regardless of color. Layers differ in deepness and transparency. Most often, seven layers are seen, although it is possible for certain people to decipher nine. There is a possibility that more layers exist, but have not currently been defined.

Each chakra corresponds to a layer of the aura and are listed from 1-7, from close to the body, moving outward. The higher the number , the higher the vibration is, this causes a current of energy that moves vertically, pulsing up and out to the perimeter of the aura. The healthier the individual, and the more open the chakras, the further that the aura can extend off of the body.

7 Aura layers explained

- Etheric Layer: This layer ranges from a ¼ in. to 2 in. away from the edge of our physical body. The etheric layer is the medium to which our own skin is affixed. It is made up of little, delicate, threads of energy that are interwoven around the body. It is almost a copy of your skin, yet it is made of energy. Flickers of energy travel through this matrix, sparkling as they flow. Many well-practiced aura viewers can see this web of energy. Beginners may only view a muted, blurry, transparent vapor, kind of like you see coming off of the ground on an extremely hot day. May people have seen it, even if they have never tried to view an aura. It can be seen as a grey to blue fog to a novice, to sparks of blue or grey light by the well-trained eye.

- The Etheric Layer is interconnected with the Root Chakra and what we experience through our five senses. This means that both physical pain and pleasure have an effect on the Etheric Body. What we eat and the way that we exercise (or lack of exercise) has an influence on it as well. The way that we feel the vibration of other's energy also takes place in the Etheric Body.

- Emotional Layer: Aptly named, this layer deals with our feelings and emotions. The Emotional Layer reaches out 1-3 in. from the physical body. It is a fluid layer that permeates all of the other layers. The unformulated flames of color do not resemble the shape of our physical body. The colors of the Emotional Body fluctuate in response to the emotion being felt at the time. The colors range from vivid with positive emotion, to muddy in response to negative emotion. It is possible to see every color in this layer, and it is usually the first layer of color that someone first learns to see.

- Intertwined with the Sacral Chakra, the Emotional Layer is connected to how we perceive ourselves, and how those perceptions make us feel. In order to keep this layer thriving, it is important to vent and feel those emotions regardless of what they are. Do not hold them in or ignore them.

- Mental Layer: Like the Etheric Layer, this layer is more defined and configured. It is found 3-8 in. away from the physical body. The Mental Layer is usually seen as yellow or gold in color, and is brightest between the head and the shoulders. The radiance of the light in this layer is brightest while concentrating and focusing on a mental task. Sometimes sparks and splotches of colors are seen are seen when one creates repetitive thought patterns. These color differences are dictated by how a person is connected emotionally to their thought processes.

- Our Mental Layer interacts with the Solar Plexus Chakra. It is interrelated with both left and right brain capabilities. The equal use of both sides of the brain, logical and imaginative, will keep the Mental Layer in good health. Daydreaming, lucid dreaming, the active use of the imagination, active learning, and the quest for knowledge are all things that we can do to achieve this well-being.

- The Mental Layer is susceptible to serious destruction if one stays in a state of negativity or cynical thinking for too long.

- Astral Layer: This vaporous layer is full of color, reaching out 1-1 ½ ft. outside the body. The Astral Layer is where we create astral cords that connect us to others, whether they are positive or negative, current or previous connections.

- The Astral Body is the area of the aura where we pick up on the vibrations of others. This layer is usually bathed in a pinkish color. The Astral Layer is a long term collection of how we feel about ourselves, on both an emotional and intellectual level . It is the connection linking experiences. The Astral Layer rules visualization, dreaming, and hallucinating. You are mentally aware of this part of yourself, but at the same time, you can still come into contact with other levels of reality.

- The Astral Layer also allows us to project, and be in two places at the same time. The Astral Layer is connected to the Heart Chakra. This connection links us to relationships with others, and how these associations have an influence on our emotions. The way to keep this layer functioning at its best is by keeping healthy and encouraging, constructive relationships with people and the world around us.

- Etheric Template Layer: This layer is located around 1 ½-2 ft. outside of the body. The Etheric Template is actually a structured blueprint/ master plan of everything that is alive on the physical level.

- It is a workable template of the Etheric Layer, a dark blue background with thin, light energy streaks. When something is wrong with the Etheric Layer, you can go into your Etheric Template to find out how to rebalance. This template is connected to the Throat Chakra, the place where noise is turned into matter. The Etheric Template is where divine will and the power of manifesting your will into existence are formed. Devine will is established by our inner, higher self and is the greatest longing for a direction in our existence that will serve a greater good.

- By aligning our free and divine wills, we can have a healthy, vivid Etheric Template Layer. When these two wills are not lined up, this layer will still have energy lines, but they will not be as plentiful nor as bright. This will cause you to feel as if you are wandering in life without purpose. By using the power of manifestation in relation to your divine and free will, you can rebalance this layer by changing your reality and existence.

- Celestial Layer: While the Etheric Layer is more of a physical form of the higher self, the Celestial Layer is the emotional form of the higher self. It is located about 2-2 ¾ ft. outside of the body. The colors in the Celestial Body are iridescent and pastel, almost like a bubble or an abalone shell. In this layer we have a connection to a higher power and generate unconditional love that attaches us to other physical beings. It generates energy, much like a star or the sun, radiating outward.

- The Celestial Body is associated with the Third Eye Chakra. It reflects our connections, on a spiritual level, with the universe. We can keep this layer healthy by practicing meditation, present moment awareness, and by pondering religion, spirituality, or the philosophies of reality and existence. The Celestial Layer is where we view the divine and spiritual nature within ourselves and in those around us. It also connected to each individual's awareness of the divine and how sensitive and open we are to the spiritual realm.

- Ketheric Template Layer: Extending 2 ½-3 ft. away from the body, this layer is where we become aware of the fact that we are one with our higher power and the universe. Its outer edge is the toughest, most durable layer.

- The Ketheric Layer is oval in shape, like an egg. Comprised of thin, pulsating golden threads, it also supplies the energy that runs through the spine, powering the entire body. The higher-self fills the Ketheric Layer and this can be seen by way of a gold glow. It is the intellectual layer of the spiritual realm. Here in the Ketheric Layer we are joined with the universal mind and are able to comprehend it, as well as being able understand past lives.

- The Ketheric Layer is intertwined with the Crown Chakra, and connects us to the universal mind. We can keep this layer healthy by understanding, and having insights regarding our place in the universal mind and our connection to the divine. This is achieved by having contact with higher power and having spiritual experiences. We can strengthen the Ketheric Layer by constantly seeking out divine wisdom, knowledge, and ideas.

Energy from others is taken into our aura. This can be good, if the other person has positive energy. Negative energies are what we need to be wary of as they can have a very detrimental effect on our aura.

We have quick, auric run-ins with people all of the time, but being around someone all of the time, or being in close proximity with a lot of people, negative energies are more easily absorbed. If you think that your aura has been disturbed and ingested negative energy there are purifying rituals that can rid your aura of the negativity.

Here are two examples of great visualization meditations that will cleanse your aura.

- The Shower:

Close your eyes. Visualize a shower: any kind, shape, size, even a waterfall. Decide on a shower that will allow you to feel comfortable and clean. Use your imagination and sense to experience everything: the smells, the texture under your feet, and the sound of the water.

Step under the water and feel the water rush over your skin. Take in everything: the temperature, the smell of the water, the rush of the cleansing water over your skin. Feel the negative energy rinsing right off of your skin as the water runs down you.

Stay in your shower until all of the negativity has washed away. Watch as the water goes down the drain or rushes away the in pool under the waterfall. The negative energy is going with it. Remain there until you are relaxed and clean.

- The Bubble:

Go to a quiet, relaxing, comfortable spot. While lying down, count to twenty, slowly with your eyes closed. Imagine, in your mind's eye, a large pink bubble quite a few feet above you.

Slowly, use all of your energy and imagination to visualize transporting all negative energy that is congesting your aura up and away from you into the bubble.

Do this for as long as long as it takes to feel released from the negativity. Once you feel the "all clear," allow the bubble, full of the negative energy, higher and higher, up into the air until you see it disappear. Now that it is gone, you are free of that negativity.

Negative human energy is not the only kind of negative energy that can mess up your aura. The negative energy in any given location can be absorbed into the aura. Auras are prone to taking on negativity from environments like: jails, graveyards, haunted locations, various types of medical facilities, locations of frequent drug use, and many more. Try to keep your time at these kinds of places short and infrequent. Use cleansing rituals after you leave. You can keep absorption to a minimum by waving your arms around, dissipating and pushing the negative energy churning around you away. Sage (the white variety) can also be used to strengthen and stimulate your own auras positive energy. Black tourmaline is also an easy way to fend off negative energy. Some people carry it in their pocket, but a fun way to keep it with you is to have a piece of jewelry that contains it.

Knowing that the physical body is related to the auric bodies, keeping the physical health in shape will also keep our aura vivid and brilliant. Just as the circulation of the physical body is detrimental to health, so is the circulation of energy important to auric health. Eating well can help certain chakras to open up. The Heart Chakra responds to dark leafy greens. Lean proteins will help to ground the Root Chakra. The Third Eye and Crown Chakras respond well to the antioxidant properties found in dark berries and dark grapes. Not only can we eat our way to physical health, we can eat our way to auric health!

One more thing you can do to keep your aura functioning at its best is to spend time in nature. Nature is full of positive energy. Spending time out doors will help to relax the body and mind, and rejuvenate the spirit. Amp up your aura and allow nature to cleanse and heal it. Even something as simple as taking a barefoot walk in the grass or dirt is very cleansing and will ground you. Relax in the ocean, let the waves crash into you. Float down a river or wade in a stream. These natural water sources have a very cleansing quality. Nature will allow you to feel free, and give you a more positive perspective, which will in turn brighten and strengthen your aura.

Cindy Walker

THE POWER OF COLORS

Auras surround the entirety of the body, but are usually easiest to see around the head and shoulder area. We will discuss the colors and their meanings based on this area of the body.

Before we investigate the actual meanings behind certain colors, here are some added tips when reading auric color:

Most auras have 1-2 principal colors. They are known as "auric pairs" and will sometimes be the person's favorite color.

The more vivid the aura, the more aware and spiritual the person most likely is.

The more evenly that the energy is spread out in the aura more likely it is that the person is in good health.

The aura is not only comprised of dominant colors. They also contain changing flickers, sparks, or flame-like flashes that come and go. These are usually contemplations, feelings, ideas, and wants.

The color of these flashes usually falls under the definitions as follows:

- Red: An aura that is principally red usually signals a person who is very concerned with material possessions and physical appearance. Flashes of red usually indicate thoughts that are material items or something physical about the body.

- Pink (a combination of purple and red): An aura that is pink, is a combination of purple (highest frequency) and red (lowest frequency). Pink auras signal a person who has a balance of materialism and spirituality. A few people may be seen with a halo that is yellow and a huge exuding pink aura. This is a very rare dominant aura color and is usually only seen as a thought, temporarily.

- Orange: An aura that has orange as its dominant color. Orange is inspirational and fascinating. People with orange auras are inspirational and authoritative. They usually have the power to control people. When orange is a dominant color, usually a gold halo can be seen, denoting a powerful spiritual instructor. An orange flicker usually represents a thought that the person is having in regard to commanding others.

- Yellow: Someone with a yellow aura is joyful, charitable, and free. A yellow halo will only be seen on a person who is a spiritual instructor, as it signals extraordinary spiritual growth. The thickness of the halo will be one inch or less. The yellow halo is an auric pair with the violet brow chakra. Those who are working to a high level of spirituality focus attention on this chakra because they are concentrating on divine thoughts. Yellow flickers of thought signal ideas and feelings of jubilation and serenity.

- Green: People who have green auras are usually healers by nature. The more dominant and clear the green aura , the more practiced or efficient the healer. Green auras usually have a "green thumb" as well and are great at gardening. Being near a green aura will bring you tranquility and peace. When you see green flashes, this signals that the person is in a position of restoration and relaxation.

- Turquoise: Auras of this color indicate that the person is a great at multitasking, high-energy, and has great organizational skills. They like to think about many things at the same time, and have great influence over others. People with turquoise auras make great supervisors in the workplace because they go over their objectives and visions, motivating their subordinates instead of just demanding compliance. Turquoise flashes and flames indicate a thought or idea related to organization or persuading others.

- Blue: People who have dominant blue auras are tranquil, well-adjusted, and sensible. They are survivalists and can go run off to live in a cave or bunker. They would be happy to live off of the land. Blue flickers usually indicate thoughts about survival and the relaxation of the nervous system. A bright, vivid blue supersedes any auric color. It is usually seen when someone is telepathically accepting or conveying communication.

- Purple: Purple is never a dominant aura color, only as flickers of thoughts. They represent exceptionally divine thoughts.

- Darker, Smokey Colors

- Brown: Worrisome, disturbing, selfish, greedy, materialistic, thoughts that oppose divinity and spirituality.

- Grey: Morbid, discouraging, and depressing thoughts. May show unclear motives or the existence of a dark side. Mustard-like: Signals discomfort, hardship, rage, or resentment.

- White: The color white signifies problems in the aura. White color is like a racket, compared to the melodious pitch that an aura should have. White indicates discord in the person.

Before a person passes away, the aura turns white. That is why, historically, death is characterized by white, instead of black.

The understanding of auric colors will help you to understand more about your true-self, and the true nature of others. In dealing with ourselves, it helps us to see areas of improvement and where we really are on our path to enlightenment. Not only that , it can be the first step in figuring out what your strong points really are and the potential to use them to the best of your ability. Not only that, but you may see an indicator for illness, or negative energy that you could have picked up from someone else, or that you have inside of yourself. When dealing with others, our understanding of auric colors can help us to enlighten others about their true nature and possible physical and emotional health concerns. It also allows us to see past fake personalities in order to determine the kinds of people we want to allow into our lives.

CAN YOU READ AURAS?

Being able to see an aura is a very practical, insightful tool. It will help you to learn more about yourself and those around you. For most people, it takes a bit of training and practice to learn how to see an aura.

There are many different approaches and tips that will allow you to train your eyes and your consciousness to make it possible. Auras can be difficult to see at first, but once you realize that you can do it, and it clicks, you will be able to repeat the process. Naturally it is easy for kids to see auras. Babies can see them as well because they have clear, balanced chakras.

There are many ways to learn how to see auras. If you are not a "natural," do not worry, with practice you can learn how to train your eyes to see them. The techniques I have listed will aid you in figuring out how. They will also help you practice and hone your skills . Some of the methods are for use on people and others for objects. Try them all and see what works best for you. For some it may take more work, but it is possible for everyone to learn how to see auras.

Reading Other People/ White Background

- Put your subject in front of a white background with nothing on it. Make sure that there are no shadows.

- Using a colored background will make it harder. Pick a spot on the person to focus on. It will allow your peripheral vision to take over.

- You will be concentrating on one spot, and this will allow the rest of your vision to relax. Indian culture suggests that you focus on the third eye, right between the eyebrows. Stare at this spot for a minute or longer, without losing focus. This will take practice.

- Every time you find your gaze moving, refocus. After a minute, become aware of your peripheral vision.

- You must do this without taking your concentration off of your focal point. This too will take practice, and if you lose your focal point, refocus and start over.

When you do this, you should notice that the border between the body and the background has a glowing color to it. It should be a color different than the rest of the backdrop.

The longer that you focus your vision, the brighter it should become. By focusing on one spot, you are increasing your visual sensitivity to the aura. You can also allow your eyes to go out of focus, if you know how. This will allow you to pick up on other visual cues you may not have noticed.

Additional tips: Once you achieve seeing the color, have your subject shift their body from side to side. You should see their aura moving as well. Do not work on focusing for too long. Only engage in the practice for a couple of minutes at a time. Let your eyes rest in between moments of focus. If you are not seeing the aura clearly, try playing your subject's favorite music. This may invigorate their aura, allowing it to be seen more clearly.

Reading Yourself/ White Background/ Hand:

- Use a white wall or a sheet of white paper. Make sure that the lighting is natural: the sun or a candle. Do not do this at night.

- Practice in a room that is shaded from direct sunlight, if it is too bright, it will not work properly.

- Hold up a hand against the white background and let your eyes relax. Focus on the tips of the fingers or allow your eyes to become out of focus (this works best for me). Slowly but surely, you will see a clear or blue-ish glow start to form around your hand.

- Keep your gaze steady, and refocus or relax again as necessary. Eventually the brightness will turn into a color.

- Decide exactly what colors you are seeing.

Extra tips: Sometimes you will see an "after image" or a negative looking effect. Do not base your auric color on this. You will be able to tell if it is a negative image if you look away from your subject matter and wherever you look you will see the same image inversely. Just like when you stare at a bright light for a long period of time and see it no matter where you look for a minute or so afterward.

Also, do not worry if you start to see the color and it disappears quickly. Blinking your eyes and loss of focus is common. Afterwards, it is helpful and fun to take a white piece of paper and draw an outline of your body. Using colored pencils, pastels, whatever you like , sketch out the colors you see. You can keep them on hand, for your own personal reference, or just to show others.

Do not get discouraged if you do not see anything right away. You have to relax, practice, and train your eyes . Try these exercises when you are relaxed and in a place free of distraction. If sunlight is not working for you, use a dark room only illuminated with candlelight.

Reading Yourself/ Mirror

- Have large mirror about four feet in front of you.

- Try to make sure that the background behind you is white.

- You should see to it that there are as few shadows as possible.

- The lighting should be constant and soft.

- Follow the same instructions above (as when you used your hand).

Do this for 10 15 minutes every day. This will help you to train your eyes to see auras.

Additional tips: Once you are able to see your inner-aura, the bluish, white glow, you can try your hand at seeing color. As in the previous exercise, place yourself in front of the mirror. Focus on seeing that same inner aura again, but now, try to concentrate on the border of that glow.

With practice, the glow will grow wider. You should be slowly able to see color start to border the edge, and it may be hazy, or dim at first. This is how you be able to see the color of the middle aura. It will take time, but step by step you should become more comfortable with it.

From here you can move on to seeing the shape of the aura. You will need all the materials in the exercises above, but this time a full length mirror would be helpful. Find the border, your white glow, and relax your vision to see the other colors. Start with your head, and when you lose focus, simply bring it back. It is a practice of refocusing your attention.

As you get more skilled, you can train your eyes to see the aura in front of the body, not only around it. Once you are focused, follow the aura from one side of the body to another. Across the top of the head is a good place to try: move from one shoulder, over the head, to the other shoulder. After you master that, try looking at the front of you, even down your torso, groin and legs.

Reading Yourself/ Fingers

- Place your hands together, press your pointer tips together. Pull them apart just a bit.

- Concentrate your gaze in between them. You are trying to focus on waves of energy passing between them, kind of like heat waves on a warm asphalt parking lot.

- Relax your vision every so often and let them go out of focus intermittently.

Another option, using your digits, stretch one of your arms out directly in front of you. Put your hand into a fist, thumb facing up. Move the thumb to eye-level. Now, concentrate you gaze on the tip. Hold your focus, without blinking for as long as possible. If performed correctly, you should be able to make out whips of energy, right there at the tip.

How to see the aura of a tree

Trees are large and produce an aura that can be huge, strong, and clearly visible. Try to do it around dawn or in the evening. Pick a tree that is tall, broad, and stands alone. Stand approximately 20 feet away from it. Focus on the tree's outline. It should be a hazy, green/ gay color. You will see this outline between the sky and the tree most often faintly at first, then once you have caught a glimpse of it, let your eyes go out of focus a bit or squint slightly. Practice for as long as you need to. You can try other trees as well.

How to see the aura of a plant

Find a plant that is still. Potted plants work well for this exercise. Find a spot to focus you attention on, either near the top or the base. Allow your eyes to relax and go out of focus. This can also be accomplished by focusing slightly beyond the plant. Slowly, the white aura of the plant should begin to appear. You may not see the same colors you would when reading a person's aura, but it is still a useful practice. It will help to train your eyes to see other auras.

Practicing Tips and Tricks

1. Practice your sensing skills. Be aware of how you feel around others. What "vibe" are they giving you? Are they pulling from your energy or adding to it? While paying attention to their energy, focus on your breathing. Note what your physical senses are telling you, how they are making your mind and body feel. Practice picturing the color this person makes you feel. You may not always be correct, but it is a great way to start sensing aura. Visualization and sensation go hand in hand.

2. Practice using your peripheral vision. This is an ability that most people have, but because we do not always use it in everyday life, it must be strengthened . It is also an area of sight that has not incurred as much damage as the rest of the eye. You can practice for a minute or so at a time by focusing sight on one spot. It will heighten your sensitivity, and you will notice a big difference in your focus in the far corners of your vision.

3. Practice with colors. Find a white solid background, like a wall, and make sure the lighting is mellow, no direct glare. Wrap a book in a bright

primary colored paper and stand it up on a table, facing you, white wall in the background. Place yourself a few feet away. Take a few cleansing breaths with your eyes closed, open them looking directly at your subject. Practice on focusing on the border of it, even a little bit past it. You should start to see a thin, glowing border. Keep your focus and you should notice it turning a greenish-yellow. This can be done with many objects and colors. It will help you train your eyes to see color that our everyday vision does not always pick up. When you lose focus during a practice such as this, do not worry, you are not doing it wrong. Stay relaxed and refocused, the more you do it the better your eyes will be at balancing themselves this way.

4. Quick fixes: honing your aura reading skills can be done all the time. There are little things you can do anywhere. Gauge the aura of a customer or co-worker. Focus on them and you may notice a difference in it as they become angry, frustrated, comfortable, or pleased. When at the beach, look at the border of the water on the horizon. The top of a crest of a crashing wave is also electrifying. Nature holds many aura-frying sights, which if we remain still and focused, can blow our minds. A simple man-made key can be a wonder. Hold it in your hand for fifteen minutes. Seal your energy into it.

Put it down, and visualize your energy in the key, you should actually be able to see your emotion fixed onto it.

Do not lose faith if you are not picking it up right away. As we move through life some people become desensitized to the process. We have to strengthen and train that ability. With any training comes practice of course! You can develop the skill to see auras, just do not give up. 15-20 minutes of practice goes a long way. Try to practice every day . The ability to sense energy takes time. As you make little steps, you will gain more confidence in your abilities. Confidence plays a huge part in the ability to see auras.

BALANCING AURAS FOR OUR PHYSICAL AND EMOTIONAL HEALTH

It is just as important for us to keep up our energy body as it is for us to keep up our physical body, yet many people neglect it. Our life energy not only affects our physical and mental health (and vice-versa), it also brings things into our life, and possibly repels others. Keeping our auras bright and healthy allows us to stay in great emotional and physical shape as well. Holistic wellness can also be thought of as holistic balance. Sadly, especially in this day and age, our life-energy body can become neglected. Now that you are aware of this, you have the power to fix it easily.

The balancing and cleansing process will not only help you to feel energized, think clearly, have control over your emotions, it will help you to deflect negative energy and pass positive energy to others. Not only is it possible to pick up negative energies from others, we can also produce it in ourselves. Negative thoughts about ourselves and past experiences create bad energy. The wrong diet, lack of exercise, or use of drugs and alcohol can also taint the aura with negative energy. This causes an imbalance or blockage in the flow of our life energy.

We know what happens when our energy is blocked or unbalanced. The aura will suffer as well as our physical being. You can become sick, feel lethargic, nervous, disheartened, or emotionally and mentally unstable. It is possible to balance and clear our flow of energy, and achieve wellness by cleansing the aura.

There are many different methods of aura cleansing available. Most are not super complicated, most are super practical and easy to use! Many of them are also beneficial to your physical health, so why not try them? Did you know that even drinking 12 glasses of spring or purified water a day will help to purify the aura? I find that using all methods in combination works well. You will enjoy engaging in these aura cleansing techniques and finding out which ones work best for you.

Bathe in sea salt.

Yes, something as simple as taking a bath in dissolved sea salt is very cleansing for your aura. We have to wash our spiritual body just like we was our physical body. This type of bath takes away negative energy while strengthening the aura. Sea salt builds a type of barrier that protects against negative energy. Sea salt is very grounding and will pull out undesirable spiritual energy from the skin. Water is purifying by nature and will cleanse our positive energy. After a sea salt bath you will be left with a protected and cleansed aura.

Different people conduct this bathing ritual in various ways. The most important things to include are a previously bathed body, sea salt, and an undisturbed period of time. 15-30 minutes is recommended. Your favorite essential oils can be added, you can burn incense, play calming music, or a guided meditation.

- Fill your bathtub with warm water and dissolve a cup or two of sea salt into it. I relax my entire body, a section at a time, bottom to top.

- Next, I visualize all of my stress, worry, self-doubt, and negative feelings brought on by others being sucked out of my body through the skin.

- Try to make sure all of your body is submerged at one point or another.

- When you are done, get out of the bath knowing you are clean and free of any negativity.

I also find that a dip in the ocean works in the same way. It is cleansing and freeing. Although you should be wary of polluted areas, as this may counteract the effect.

Light

Light visualization is easy to do. I prefer to use this method out in the sunlight, to double the effect, but it can be done indoors as well.

- Lie down in a comfortable place.

- Take a few cleansing breaths and close your eyes.

- When you are completely relaxed, visualize a white light above you. I use the sunlight that permeates my eyelids, but either will do.

- Feel the light come into your body, filling every inch of it. As it engulfs the body, imagine it taking the place of negative energy.

- Imagine the light cleansing and repairing the entirety of your body. Relish in the moment.

- After you have done this for a while, visualize extending the light outside of your body. See it pushing out all negative energy. Feel all of your negative energy leaving your body and moving far away from you.

The light has now restored your energy and replaced all negativity.

Deep Breathing

Deep breathing is very cleansing for your aura. This one is simple by nature, but is sometimes tricky to get the hang of.

- The more you practice, the easier it will become. Once a day, find a quiet spot where you will be undisturbed. At first do this exercise in 5-10 minute increments and then work up to half hour sessions.

- You should sit comfortably and close your eyes. Start by inhaling for four seconds. Exhale for four seconds. Each time you inhale feel the breath penetrate deep down into your stomach.

- Concentrate on your breathing as you to this. You are focusing attention only on the inhale and the exhale of your breath. Every time you get distracted, simply redirect your attention to your breath. Continue this process until you are fully relaxed.

- After a few minutes, each time you inhale imagine that you are inhaling a white, glowing, flow of energy. As the breath enters your body, imagine that you are filled with a glowing white light.

- Feel the light restoring your body and your energy.

- Upon exhaling, see your breath coming out as dark negative energy.

- Experience the feeling of relief as you push out negative energy. Each time your lungs empty, experience a peace knowing that your energy is balanced.

Use a sage stick for smudging away negative energy.

It is an ancient cleansing process that sounds "hocus-pocus-y," but really works.

- Simply purchase one at a new age or health food store.

- Light one end of the stick.

- When you see a flame, blow it out and it should begin to smolder.

- Swirl stick around yourself as the smoke encircles you.

- The smoke will rid you of bad energy.

Crystals work well to cleanse the aura and protect it.

There is much to learn about the science behind crystals, how to use them in healing, and how they protect the aura. Let me give you a few basic ways that a beginner such as yourself can easily use crystals for cleansing . When in doubt, or for more complicated crystal usage consult a professional.

- One good thing that crystals are great for is to protect a cleansed aura from negative energy. Black Tourmaline can be carried with you. Rose Quartz is good as well because it substitutes negative energy for positive energy.

- Labradorite keeps people from sucking away at your positive energy. It will protect your aura from being leeched off of by others.

- Amethyst, Bloodstone, Citrine, and Quartz are all great cleansing stones.

- You can use these stones by carrying them on your person, waving them around you through your aura, wearing them on a piece of jewelry, or putting one next to your bed.

- You can also meditate with a crystal.

- Here is an easy way for a beginner to practice an aura cleanse. Find a quiet place and lie down. Practice some deep breathing mediation for a few minutes with your crystal placed on your third eye chakra. Now visualize a white glow coming from the crystal. Allow the light to course through your body, and then around it. Let the light purify your aura, as it encircles your body in a cleansing glow. Do this until you feel refreshed and clean.

Essential oils are fabulous aura cleansers and are very easy to use. You can have them mixed professionally, or choose a single oil to use on your own.

Common cleansing oils are: lime, juniper, cinnamon, cypress, and lemon.

- Make your own aura misting cleanser by using a clean spray bottle, filling it with a cup of spring water, and adding a couple of drops of the essential oil of your choice. Mix it will and spray yourself!

- You can add a few drops of essential oils to a cleansing bath. Easier still, using your finger, put a few drops at your neck and the inside of your wrists and ankles. Inhale the aroma left on your fingers with slow deep breaths while you imagine your aura brightening as you inhale, and negativity exiting with your exhale.

Those are many practical, everyday ways you can easily cleanse your aura. How can you tell if your methods work? You will feel cleansed, at ease, of sound mind, and positive... back to yourself.

You do not have to do them every day, but consistency is key. Find what works best for you. If you do not feel like these methods are working for you. I encourage you to see someone who specializes in aura or energy healing.

Living a peaceful and balanced life

Life is a journey that we are all on. In order to make the most of it, it is of the utmost importance to live holistically balanced in order to achieve holistic wellness. This is not only important for our own personal journey , happiness, spiritual health, and physical wellbeing, it is detrimental to those around us.

The energy of the universe is alive in all of us, and we are alive in it. Everyone plays a part in each other's existence. If you want to be a beneficial element, radiating healthy, vibrant energy, it is important to learn how to understand and feel our own energy in order to see how it has an effect on our own health, circumstances, and relationships.

Now that you know the basics on aura and energy I urge you to get started! You see the need for holistic wellness and energy balance in your life and how necessary it is. Your energy must be balanced and your aura bright and healthy in order to maintain healthy meaningful relationships. Use the tools and information provided to enrich your life in all areas.

ABOUT THE AUTHOR

Cindy Walker is a Hypnotherapist, Life Coach and Spiritual Medium. She helps people heal, transform and awaken to their inner purpose. Her own healing journey lead her to a deeper understanding of holographic healing through meditation and working with benevolent Entities from beyond the veil.